THE HERBAL MEDICINE 2024

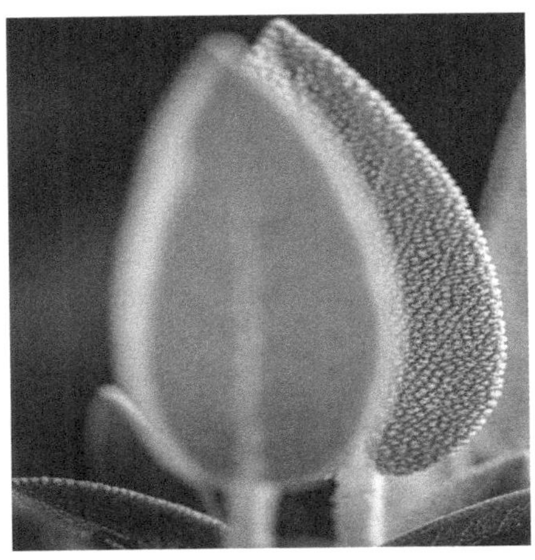

Embarking on a Journey of Plant Wellness

Ruth Larry

Table of contents

Introduction

In 2024, herbal medicine continues to evolve as a prominent aspect of holistic healthcare, blending traditional wisdom with modern scientific advancements. As society increasingly seeks natural alternatives and integrative approaches to wellness, herbal medicine occupies a central role in preventative care and therapeutic interventions. This resurgence in interest stems from a growing appreciation for the holistic principles of herbalism, which emphasize the interconnectedness of mind, body, and environment.

Advancements in research and technology have propelled herbal medicine into the forefront of modern healthcare. Scientists are continually exploring the pharmacological properties of botanicals, uncovering new compounds and mechanisms of action. This intersection of traditional knowledge and cutting-edge science has led to the development of standardized herbal extracts, refined formulations, and evidence-based practices.

Furthermore, the accessibility of information through digital platforms has empowered individuals to explore herbal remedies and self-care practices. Online resources, educational courses, and community forums facilitate the sharing of knowledge and experiences, democratizing healthcare and fostering a culture of empowerment and self-reliance.

In addition to its therapeutic benefits, herbal medicine also plays a crucial role in sustainable healthcare and environmental conservation. By promoting the cultivation of medicinal plants and supporting local growers, herbalism fosters a deeper connection to the earth and promotes biodiversity. Moreover, the emphasis on natural remedies reduces reliance on synthetic pharmaceuticals, minimizing environmental impact and contributing to a more sustainable healthcare system.

As we navigate the complexities of modern life, herbal medicine offers a holistic approach to wellness that honors the innate wisdom of nature. Whether used as a complement to conventional treatments or as a primary form of care, herbal medicine continues to inspire hope and healing in individuals and communities worldwide.

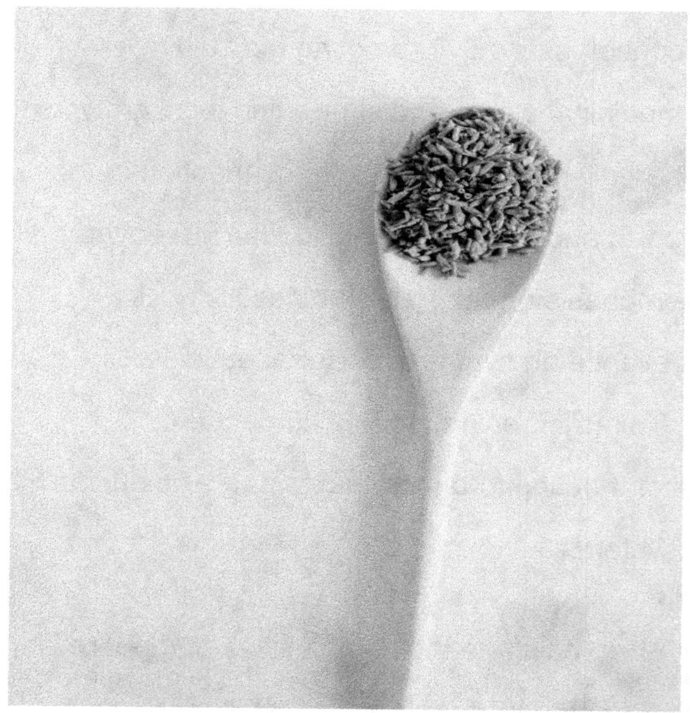

Chapter One

Understanding the principles of herbalism

Understanding the principles of herbalism is fundamental to harnessing the power of medicinal plants effectively. Here are some key principles:

1. **Holism:** Herbalism views the body as a holistic system, interconnected with the mind and spirit. Rather than treating symptoms in isolation, herbalists aim to address underlying imbalances and promote overall wellness.
2. **Individualization:** Herbal remedies are tailored to each person's unique constitution, health history, and specific needs. What works for one individual may not work for another, emphasizing the importance of personalized treatment.

3. **Vitalism:** Herbalism often incorporates the concept of vitalism, which recognizes the body's innate ability to heal itself when supported with the right tools and conditions. Herbal remedies are seen as catalysts for the body's own healing processes.

4. **Doctrine of Signatures:** This ancient concept suggests that the appearance of a plant, such as its color, shape, or habitat, provides clues to its medicinal properties. While not strictly scientific, the doctrine of signatures can offer insights into a plant's potential uses.

5. **Energetics:** Herbalism considers the energetic qualities of plants, including their taste, temperature, and affinity for certain organs or systems in the body. These energetic properties inform herbalists' choices in selecting herbs and formulating remedies.

6. **Prevention and Balance:** Herbal medicine emphasizes prevention and the maintenance of balance within the body. By supporting overall health and addressing imbalances early on, herbal remedies can help prevent illness and promote vitality.

7. **Respect for Nature:** Herbalists often advocate for sustainable harvesting practices, ethical wildcrafting, and cultivation methods that honor the Earth and its ecosystems. Respecting nature ensures the availability of medicinal plants for future generations.

By understanding and applying these principles, herbalists can effectively harness the healing potential of plants while promoting holistic well-being and harmony with nature.

Historical perspectives

Historical perspectives and cultural context play a significant role in shaping the practice of herbalism around the world. Throughout history, medicinal plants have been a cornerstone of healthcare in diverse cultures, with each civilization contributing its unique knowledge and practices to the rich tapestry of herbal medicine.

Ancient Civilizations: The use of medicinal plants dates back thousands of years, with evidence of herbal remedies found in ancient Egyptian papyri, Mesopotamian clay tablets, and Chinese texts like the Huangdi Neijing. These early civilizations relied heavily on plants for healing, often integrating herbal remedies into religious rituals and everyday life.

Traditional Systems of Medicine: Many cultures developed sophisticated systems of herbal medicine, such as Ayurveda in India, Traditional Chinese Medicine (TCM) in China, and Indigenous healing traditions practiced by Native American, African, and South American cultures. These systems are deeply rooted in cultural beliefs, spirituality, and a holistic understanding of health and illness.

Herbalism in the Middle Ages: During the Middle Ages in Europe, herbalism flourished as monasteries became centers of herbal knowledge and cultivation. Herbalists like Hildegard von Bingen and Nicholas Culpeper documented the medicinal properties of plants and their use in treating various ailments.

Colonialism and Global Exchange: The age of exploration and colonialism facilitated the exchange of plants and knowledge between cultures, leading to the globalization of herbal medicine. European explorers brought back exotic plants from distant lands, while indigenous healing practices influenced European herbalism.

Modern Herbalism: In the 19th and 20th centuries, the rise of scientific inquiry and pharmaceutical medicine led to a decline in traditional herbal practices in the Western world. However, there has been a resurgence of interest in herbalism in recent decades, fueled by a desire for natural alternatives, sustainability, and cultural preservation.

Cultural Diversity and Adaptation: Today, herbal medicine reflects a diverse array of cultural influences and practices. Traditional herbal knowledge is passed down through generations within families and communities, preserving unique regional traditions and wisdom. Moreover, immigrants and diaspora communities contribute to the global exchange of herbal knowledge, enriching the practice of herbalism with new perspectives and ingredients.

Understanding the historical and cultural context of herbalism provides insight into its evolution, diversity, and enduring relevance in modern healthcare. It also highlights the importance of cultural sensitivity and respectful engagement with traditional knowledge systems.

Importance of plant medicine in modern health

The importance of plant medicine in modern health is increasingly recognized, as it offers a holistic and sustainable approach to well-being. The following are salient features emphasizing its importance:

1. **Natural Healing Agents:**
   - Plant medicines harness the therapeutic properties of naturally

occurring compounds found in plants. These compounds, such as alkaloids, flavonoids, and essential oils, often exhibit healing properties without the synthetic elements present in some pharmaceuticals.

2. **Holistic Wellness:**

    o Plant medicine emphasizes a holistic approach, addressing not just symptoms but the underlying causes of health issues. This aligns with the modern understanding that well-being involves the integration of physical, mental, and emotional health.

3. **Reduced Side Effects:**

- Many plant medicines offer therapeutic benefits with fewer side effects compared to synthetic drugs. This is especially relevant as people seek alternatives that minimize adverse reactions while promoting healing.

4. **Complementary to Conventional Treatments:**

   - Plant medicine often complements conventional medical treatments. Integrative approaches recognize the synergies between plant-based remedies and pharmaceutical interventions, enhancing overall health outcomes.

5. **Preventive Health Practices:**

- Incorporating plant medicines into daily routines can contribute to preventive health practices. Herbal teas, dietary supplements, and herbal remedies are often used to support the immune system, reduce stress, and maintain overall vitality.

6. **Cultural and Traditional Wisdom:**

   - Drawing on the wisdom of traditional healing practices, plant medicine respects diverse cultural approaches to health. Integrating this knowledge into modern health practices fosters cultural sensitivity and inclusivity.

7. **Sustainability and Environmental Consciousness:**

- Plant medicine aligns with the growing emphasis on sustainable and eco-friendly practices. Responsibly sourcing and cultivating medicinal plants contribute to environmental conservation and biodiversity.

8. Personalized Health Care:

- Recognizing individual differences, plant medicine allows for personalized health care. Tailoring remedies to an individual's unique needs and constitution contributes to more effective and personalized healing experiences.

9. Psychological Well-being:

- A growing body of research suggests that exposure to nature and plant-based environments positively influences mental health. Plant medicines, through aromatherapy and other applications, contribute to stress reduction and psychological well-being.

10. Accessibility and Affordability:

- Many plant medicines are accessible and affordable, making them a viable option for individuals seeking cost-effective and readily available health solutions.

As modern health care continues to evolve, the integration of plant medicine offers a holistic and sustainable pathway towards improved health outcomes, emphasizing the

interconnectedness of human well-being with
the natural world.

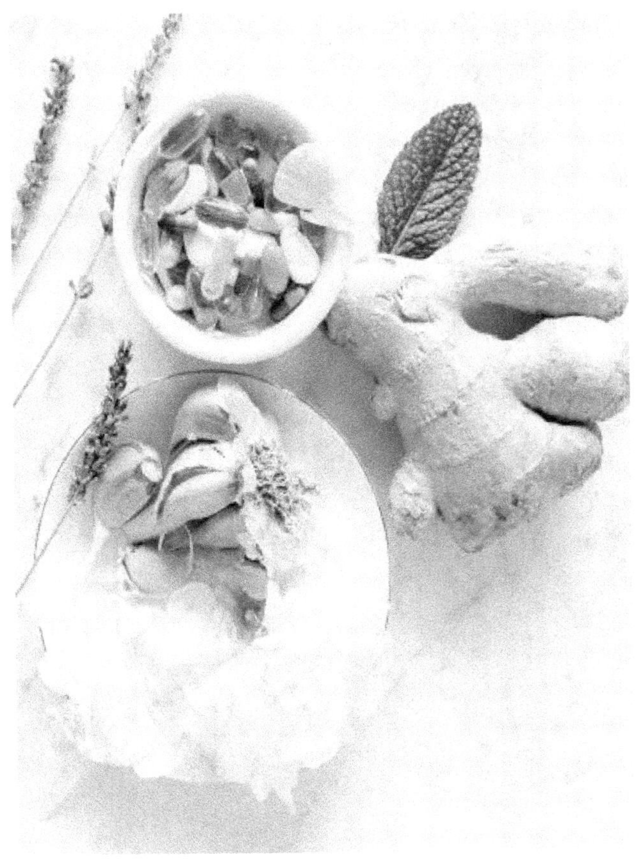

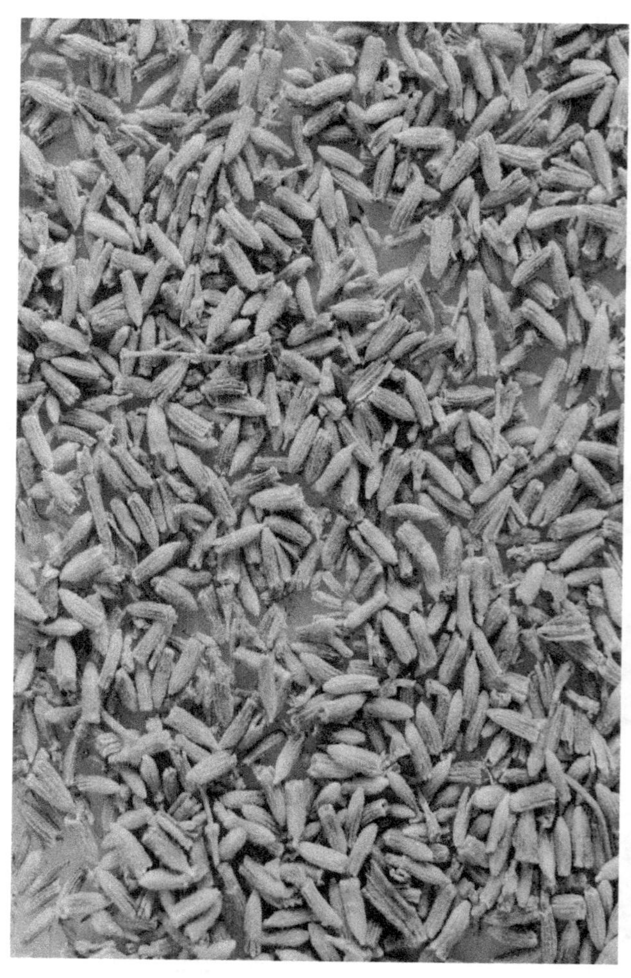

22

Chapter Two

Exploring Plant-based Remedies

Exploring Plant-Based Remedies: A Journey into Natural Healing

Embarking on the exploration of plant-based remedies is a transformative journey that invites individuals to reconnect with the healing power of nature. This endeavor involves understanding, selecting, and utilizing botanical treasures for various health and well-being purposes.

1. **Understanding the Botanical Realm:**

- Delve into the diverse world of medicinal plants, learning about their botanical classifications, growth habitats, and the bioactive compounds they contain.

- Grasp the principles of phytochemistry, unraveling the intricate web of alkaloids, terpenes, flavonoids, and other constituents that contribute to the therapeutic potential of plants.

2. **Traditional Wisdom and Indigenous Knowledge:**

- Explore the wealth of traditional healing practices from cultures around the world. Indigenous knowledge offers insights into the historical and cultural significance of specific plants for medicinal purposes.

- Understand the rituals, ceremonies, and holistic approaches embedded in traditional plant-based remedies.

3. **Herbal Teas and Infusions:**

- Dive into the world of herbal teas, discovering the unique flavors and healing properties of plants like chamomile, peppermint, and ginger.
- Learn the art of crafting herbal infusions, exploring blends that cater to individual health needs and preferences.

4. **Essential Oils and Aromatherapy:**

- Uncover the aromatic wonders of essential oils and their therapeutic

applications in aromatherapy. Explore
how plant essences can influence
mood, alleviate stress, and contribute to
overall well-being.

- Understand proper dilution methods and
safe practices for using essential oils
effectively.

5. Tinctures, Extracts, and Elixirs:

- Navigate the world of tinctures and
extracts, exploring the process of
preserving and concentrating plant
compounds in alcohol or other solvents.
- Create personalized elixirs by combining
potent plant extracts for targeted health
benefits.

6. Cultivating Medicinal Gardens:

- Embrace the hands-on experience of cultivating a medicinal garden. Learn the art of selecting, planting, and caring for medicinal plants in both indoor and outdoor settings.

- Discover the joy of harvesting fresh herbs and plants for immediate use in teas, tinctures, or culinary applications.

7. **DIY Plant Medicine Recipes:**

- Engage in the creation of do-it-yourself plant-based remedies. From soothing balms to herbal salves and digestive tonics, explore a spectrum of recipes that cater to specific health concerns.

- Understand the importance of proper dosage and consistency in preparing and administering homemade remedies.

8. Integrating Plant Remedies with Conventional Approaches:

- Explore the synergies between plant-based remedies and conventional medical treatments. Recognize situations where a complementary approach may enhance overall health outcomes.
- Consult with healthcare professionals when integrating plant medicine into a broader health care plan.

9. Nurturing Mind-Body Connection:

- Recognize the interconnectedness of mental, emotional, and physical well-being through plant-based therapies. Explore mindfulness practices, herbal rituals, and botanical experiences that contribute to holistic health.

10. Sustainable Practices and Ethical Harvesting:

- Emphasize the importance of ethical harvesting and sustainable practices to preserve plant biodiversity and ecosystems.

- Cultivate a mindset of environmental stewardship, ensuring that the exploration of plant-based remedies aligns with principles of conservation and respect for nature.

Exploring plant-based remedies is not just a pursuit of natural healing but a reconnection with the intricate and harmonious relationship between humans and the botanical world. It is

a journey that fosters empowerment,
self-discovery, and a deep appreciation for the
healing gifts nature provides.

Foundations of Herbalism

In the vast realm of natural medicine, medicinal
plants stand as time-tested allies, offering a
plethora of therapeutic compounds to support
human health and well-being. This
comprehensive overview delves into the
diverse world of medicinal plants, exploring
their classifications, historical significance, and
the wealth of bioactive compounds they harbor.

I. **Taxonomy and Classification:**

- *Botanical Families:* Medicinal plants span various botanical families, from Asteraceae to Lamiaceae, each contributing unique healing properties.
- *Herbaceous and Woody Plants:* Understanding the distinctions between herbaceous and woody plants provides insights into their growth patterns and cultivation requirements.

II. **Historical Significance:**

- *Ancient Herbalism:* Medicinal plants have been integral to the healing practices of ancient civilizations, documented in texts like the Ebers Papyrus (Egypt) and the herbal traditions of China and India.

- *Herbals of the Middle Ages:* The medieval period witnessed the compilation of herbals, such as "De Materia Medica" by Dioscorides, serving as foundational texts for herbal knowledge.

III. **Global Diversity of Medicinal Flora:**

- *Cultural Variations:* Different cultures have their own repertoire of medicinal plants, influenced by geography, climate, and traditional knowledge. Examples include ginseng in East Asia, neem in India, and eucalyptus in Australia.
- *Indigenous Wisdom:* Indigenous communities worldwide possess invaluable knowledge about local flora,

contributing to a rich tapestry of plant-based healing practices.

IV. Bioactive Compounds and Phytochemistry:

- *Alkaloids:* Many medicinal plants contain alkaloids with diverse pharmacological effects, such as morphine in opium poppy and quinine in cinchona.
- *Flavonoids:* These compounds, found in fruits, vegetables, and herbs, exhibit antioxidant and anti-inflammatory properties, contributing to the health benefits of plants.
- *Terpenes:* Aromatic compounds like essential oils are rich in terpenes, influencing the fragrance and therapeutic effects of medicinal plants.

V. **Traditional Uses and Folk Medicine**:

- *Herbal Traditions:* Traditional healing systems, including Ayurveda, Traditional Chinese Medicine, and Native American medicine, have long relied on the medicinal properties of plants.
- *Folk Remedies:* Folk medicine practices passed down through generations often involve the use of local plants for common ailments and health maintenance.

VI. **Pharmacological Research and Modern Validation:**

- *Scientific Exploration:* Advances in pharmacological research have led to the isolation and identification of active compounds in medicinal plants.

- *Clinical Studies:* Modern science validates traditional uses through clinical studies, confirming the efficacy of plant-based remedies for conditions ranging from pain management to immune support.

VII. Common Medicinal Plants and Their Uses:

- *Echinacea:* Known for immune support.
- *Ginger:* Used for digestive health and anti-inflammatory effects.
- Turmeric: Well known for its antioxidant and anti-inflammatory qualities.
- *Aloe Vera:* Applied topically for skin conditions.

- *Peppermint:* Utilized for digestive relief and respiratory support.

VIII. **Cultivation and Harvesting Practices:**

- *Sustainable Cultivation:* The importance of cultivating medicinal plants sustainably to ensure their availability for future generations.
- *Harvesting Guidelines:* Best practices for harvesting, preserving, and storing medicinal plants to maintain their potency and efficacy.

IX. **Integration with Modern Healthcare:**

- *Complementary Approaches:* The integration of medicinal plants with

conventional medicine, emphasizing a
holistic and complementary approach to
health care.

- *Phytomedicine:* The emergence of
phytomedicine as a field that explores
the medicinal properties of plants within
a scientific framework.

X. **Future Trends and Innovations:**

- *Research and Development:* Ongoing
research on novel medicinal plant
compounds and their potential
applications.
- *Technology and Extraction Methods:*
Innovations in technology and extraction
methods to enhance the bioavailability
of plant constituents.

In conclusion, the overview of medicinal plants unveils a vast and intricate world of natural healing. From ancient herbal traditions to modern scientific validation, medicinal plants continue to play a pivotal role in promoting health and offering a harmonious synergy between humans and the botanical realm.

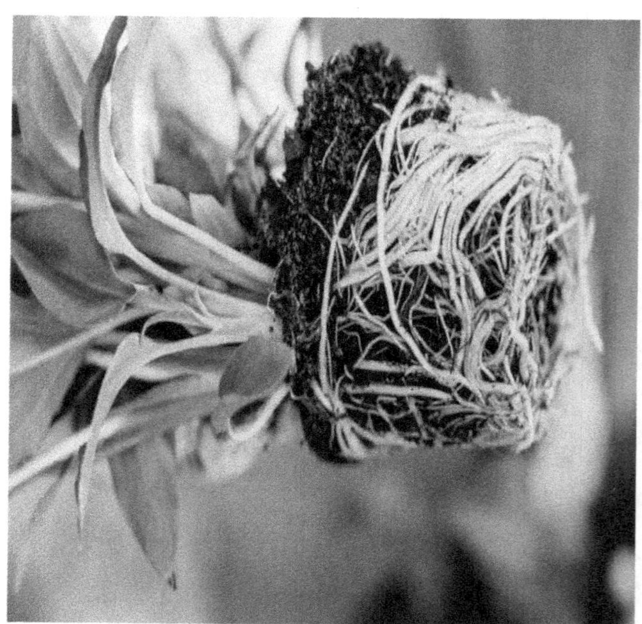

Chapter Three

Pharmacology of medicinal plants

The pharmacology of medicinal plants encompasses the study of the chemical constituents, pharmacological actions, and therapeutic uses of plant-derived compounds for treating various health conditions. This multidisciplinary field integrates principles of pharmacognosy, phytochemistry, pharmacology, and traditional medicine to understand the complex interactions between plants and the human body.

Chemical Constituents: Medicinal plants produce a vast array of bioactive compounds, including alkaloids, flavonoids, terpenoids, phenolics, glycosides, and polysaccharides. These compounds are responsible for the plants' therapeutic effects and often interact synergistically to produce a holistic healing response.

Pharmacological Actions: Medicinal plants exhibit diverse pharmacological actions, ranging from anti-inflammatory and antioxidant properties to antimicrobial, analgesic, immunomodulatory, and neuroprotective effects. These actions are mediated by the plant's bioactive compounds, which target specific molecular pathways and physiological processes in the body.

Mechanisms of Action: The mechanisms of action of plant-derived compounds are complex and multifaceted. They may act by modulating enzyme activity, receptor binding, signal transduction pathways, gene expression, and cellular signaling cascades.

For example, flavonoids exert antioxidant effects by scavenging free radicals and inhibiting oxidative stress, while alkaloids may interact with neurotransmitter receptors to modulate pain perception.

Bioavailability and Metabolism: The bioavailability of plant-derived compounds can vary widely depending on factors such as solubility, stability, absorption, distribution, metabolism, and excretion. Some compounds may undergo extensive metabolism in the liver, leading to the formation of active metabolites with enhanced bioactivity. Understanding the pharmacokinetics of medicinal plants is essential for optimizing their therapeutic efficacy and safety.

Synergy and Polypharmacy: Medicinal plants often contain multiple bioactive compounds that act synergistically to produce enhanced therapeutic effects. This concept of synergy is central to traditional herbal medicine, where whole plant extracts are used to harness the collective power of multiple constituents. Polypharmacy, the use of multiple herbs in combination, is another common practice in herbalism aimed at targeting multiple pathways and addressing complex health conditions.

Standardization and Quality Control: Standardization of herbal extracts is essential for ensuring consistency and potency across different batches of herbal products. Quality control measures, such as chromatographic fingerprinting, quantification of marker compounds, and testing for contaminants, help guarantee the safety, efficacy, and reproducibility of herbal medicines.

In conclusion, the pharmacology of medicinal plants is a dynamic and complex field that continues to uncover the therapeutic potential of nature's pharmacy. By elucidating the chemical composition, pharmacological actions, and mechanisms of action of plant-derived compounds, researchers can harness the healing power of medicinal plants to develop effective and evidence-based herbal therapies for promoting health and well-being.

Traditional Healings Practices

Traditional Healing Practices: A Tapestry of Cultural Wellness

Traditional healing practices are integral to diverse cultures worldwide, representing a holistic approach to health that encompasses the physical, mental, and spiritual dimensions of well-being. These practices, rooted in centuries-old wisdom, reflect a deep connection between communities and the natural world. Explore the rich tapestry of traditional healing, where rituals, herbal remedies, and spiritual guidance converge to foster balance and harmony.

I. Holistic Foundations:

- *Mind-Body-Spirit Connection:* Traditional
  healing views health holistically,
  acknowledging the interconnectedness
  of the mind, body, and spirit.
- *Energetic Balance:* Practices often seek
  to restore balance within the body's
  energetic systems, addressing
  imbalances that may manifest as illness.

II. **Indigenous Knowledge:**

- *Cultural Diversity:* Indigenous
  communities globally contribute unique
  healing practices shaped by their
  specific cultural, environmental, and
  historical contexts.
- *Oral Traditions:* Traditional healing
  knowledge is often passed down
  through oral traditions, emphasizing the

importance of storytelling and community wisdom.

III. **Rituals and Ceremonies:**

- *Sacred Practices:* Rituals and ceremonies play a crucial role in traditional healing. These practices are often deeply intertwined with spirituality and a connection to the divine or the natural world.
- *Cleansing and Purification:* Rituals involving smudging, bathing, or specific cleansing ceremonies aim to purify the individual's energy and restore harmony.

IV. **Herbal Medicine and Plant Wisdom:**

- *Sacred Plants:* Many traditional healing systems rely on the medicinal properties of sacred plants. These may include herbs, roots, and other botanicals with specific healing properties.

- *Eco-spirituality:* The use of plants goes beyond physical healing, encompassing a spiritual relationship with nature. Sustainable and respectful harvesting practices are often emphasized.

V. **Traditional Chinese Medicine (TCM):**

- *Acupuncture and Meridian Theory:* TCM employs acupuncture to balance the body's vital energy (Qi) through meridians. Herbal remedies, often prescribed in formulations, aim to restore harmony.

- *Yin-Yang Philosophy:* TCM's foundational philosophy of Yin and Yang informs the diagnosis and treatment of health imbalances.

VI. **Ayurveda in India:**

- *Doshas and Elemental Balance:* Ayurveda categorizes individuals into doshas (Vata, Pitta, Kapha) representing the balance of elements. Treatment involves lifestyle adjustments, dietary recommendations, and herbal remedies.
- *Panchakarma:* Ayurvedic detoxification practices, known as Panchakarma, aim to cleanse and rejuvenate the body.

VII. **Shamanic Healing:**

- *Spiritual Intermediaries:* Shamans act as intermediaries between the spiritual and physical realms. Healing ceremonies often involve trance, journeying, and communication with spirits.
- *Soul Retrieval:* Shamanic practices may include soul retrieval ceremonies to restore lost aspects of an individual's soul for holistic healing.

VIII. African Traditional Healing:

- *Ancestral Connections:* African traditional healing often emphasizes a connection with ancestors for guidance and support.
- *Divination:* Divination practices, such as reading bones or consulting oracles, are

used for diagnosis and treatment planning.

IX. Native American Medicine:

- *Medicine Wheels and Sacred Circles:* Indigenous peoples in North America use ceremonial circles and medicine wheels for healing rituals and connection to the natural world.
- *Herbal Knowledge:* Native American traditional healers rely on plant wisdom for various remedies, considering the spiritual significance of each plant.

X. Modern Integration and Challenges:

- *Integration with Modern Medicine:* Traditional healing practices are increasingly recognized for their complementary role in modern healthcare.
- *Cultural Challenges:* Preserving and respecting traditional healing practices face challenges from cultural appropriation, globalization, and encroachment on indigenous lands.

In essence, traditional healing practices represent a profound wisdom that transcends generations. They serve as a testament to the resilience of cultural knowledge, offering valuable insights into holistic well-being and the interconnectedness of humanity with the spiritual and natural realms.

Ethnobotany and Indigenous Knowledge

Ethnobotany and Indigenous Knowledge: Nurturing the Wisdom of Nature and Culture

I. Definition and Scope:

- *Ethnobotany Defined:* Ethnobotany is the interdisciplinary study that explores the dynamic relationship between plants and people, emphasizing how various cultures utilize plants for medicinal, ritual, and practical purposes.

- *Cultural Ecology:* The scope extends beyond plant identification, encompassing the cultural, ecological, and historical dimensions of plant use.

II. **Indigenous Knowledge Systems**:

- *Embedded Wisdom:* Indigenous knowledge systems are repositories of wisdom passed down through generations, encapsulating the intimate relationship between indigenous communities and their natural environments.
- *Oral Traditions:* Indigenous knowledge is often transmitted orally, emphasizing storytelling, rituals, and practical experiences as key educational tools.

III. **Medicinal Plant Use:**

- *Diverse Healing Traditions:* Indigenous communities worldwide have developed extensive knowledge of medicinal plants, using them to treat a wide array of ailments.

- *Spiritual Significance:* Medicinal plant use often has spiritual dimensions, with plants considered not just as remedies but as entities with profound spiritual connections.

IV. Sustainable Practices:

- *Harvesting and Conservation:* Indigenous communities practice sustainable harvesting, ensuring the long-term availability of medicinal plants.
- *Biodiversity Stewardship:* Traditional ecological knowledge contributes to biodiversity conservation, with indigenous communities often serving as stewards of their ecosystems.

V. Rituals and Ceremonies:

- *Sacred Plants:* Ethnobotany reveals the integral role of plants in indigenous rituals and ceremonies, where certain plants hold sacred significance.
- *Cultural Identity:* Plants are central to maintaining cultural identity, connecting individuals to their heritage through ceremonial practices.

VI. Food and Nutrition:

- *Culinary Traditions:* Ethnobotanical studies highlight the diverse use of plants in indigenous diets, reflecting unique culinary traditions and nutritional practices.

- *Traditional Farming Methods:*
  Indigenous knowledge contributes to
  sustainable agricultural practices,
  including traditional farming methods
  that promote biodiversity.

VII. Environmental Adaptation:

- *Local Ecological Knowledge:* Indigenous
  communities possess profound insights
  into local ecosystems, adapting to
  environmental changes based on their
  knowledge of plant and animal
  behaviors.
- *Climate Resilience:* Ethnobotanical
  knowledge aids in climate resilience, as
  indigenous practices often involve an
  understanding of seasonal variations
  and adaptive strategies.

VIII. Challenges and Conservation:

- *Cultural Erosion:* The transmission of indigenous knowledge faces challenges from cultural erosion, globalization, and external influences.
- *Conservation Initiatives:* Collaborative efforts between indigenous communities, researchers, and conservation organizations aim to protect both traditional knowledge and the biodiversity linked to it.

IX. Collaboration and Recognition:

- *Respectful Partnerships:* Ethnobotanists engage in collaborative research with indigenous communities, fostering respectful partnerships that acknowledge the value of indigenous knowledge.

- *Recognition and Rights:* Acknowledging and respecting indigenous intellectual property rights is crucial in preserving both cultural heritage and biodiversity.

X. Future Prospects:

- *Education and Empowerment:* Empowering indigenous communities through education and supporting the transmission of traditional knowledge ensures the continuity of ethnobotanical wisdom.
- *Innovation and Integration:* Ethnobotany continues to evolve, integrating indigenous knowledge with modern

scientific approaches for sustainable
and culturally sensitive solutions.

In essence, ethnobotany serves as a bridge
between scientific inquiry and indigenous
knowledge, recognizing the invaluable
contributions of diverse cultures to our
understanding of the intricate relationships
between humans and the plant kingdom.

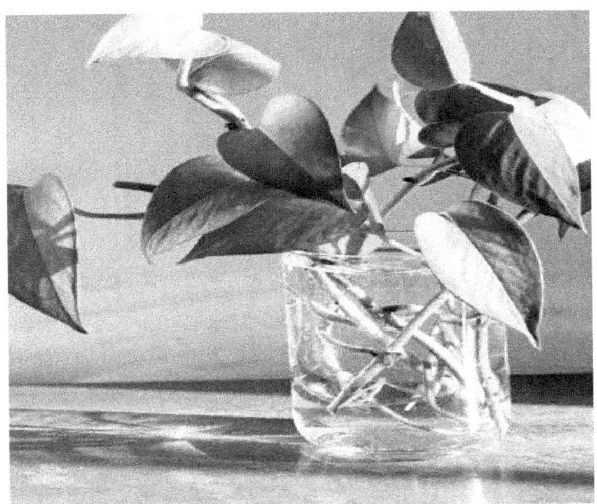

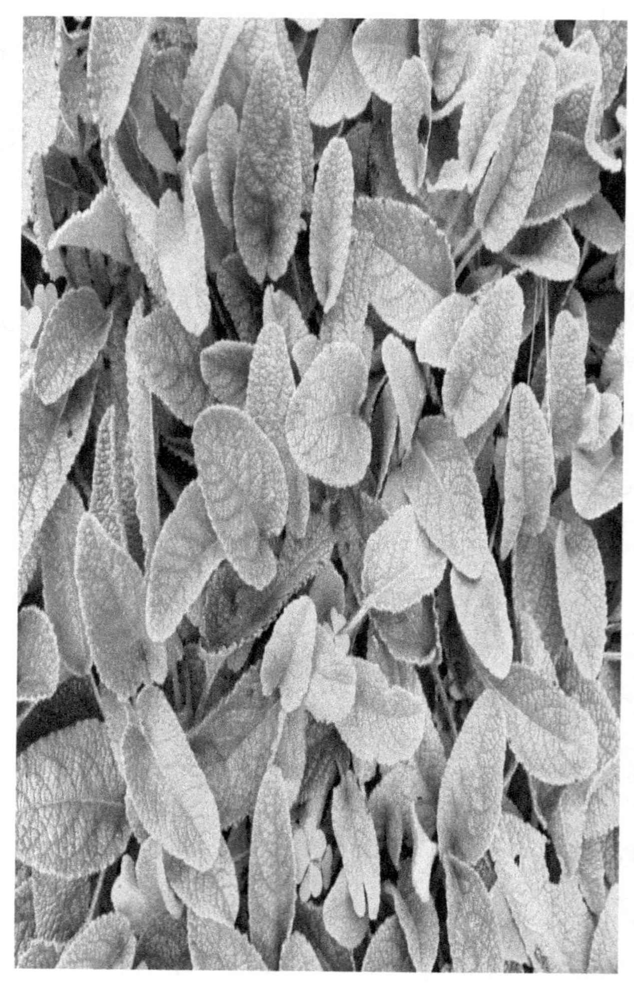

Chapter Four

Types of herbal medicines

Herbal medicine encompasses a diverse array of remedies derived from botanical sources. Here are some common types of herbal medicines:

1. **Herbal Teas and Infusions:**
   - Herbal teas are made by steeping plant materials such as leaves, flowers, or roots in hot water. They are often consumed for their therapeutic properties, including relaxation, digestion support, and immune system boost.

2. Tinctures and Extracts:

- Tinctures are concentrated liquid extracts of medicinal plants, typically made by soaking the plant material in alcohol or glycerin. They are administered in small doses and are known for their potency and shelf stability.

3. Essential Oils and Aromatherapy:

- Essential oils are highly concentrated plant extracts obtained through distillation or expression. They are used in aromatherapy, where the inhalation or topical application of essential oils can promote relaxation, mood enhancement, and various health benefits.

4. Herbal Salves and Balms:

- Herbal salves and balms are topical preparations made by infusing plant materials into oils or fats, often mixed with beeswax for consistency. They are applied to the skin for their soothing, moisturizing, and healing properties.

5. Capsules and Tablets:

- Plant-based capsules and tablets contain powdered or encapsulated forms of medicinal plants. They offer a convenient and standardized way to consume plant medicines, particularly for those who prefer a more controlled dosage.

6. Poultices and Compresses:

- Poultices are moistened plant materials applied directly to the skin to alleviate inflammation, pain, or promote wound healing. Compresses involve soaking a cloth in a herbal infusion and applying it to the affected area.

7. Herbal Baths and Soaks:

- Herbal baths and soaks involve adding medicinal plants, such as herbs or essential oils, to bathwater for their therapeutic effects. They can help relax muscles, soothe skin conditions, and promote overall relaxation.

8. Dietary Supplements:

- Plant-based dietary supplements come in various forms, including

capsules, powders, and liquid
extracts. They provide
concentrated doses of specific
plant compounds known for their
health-promoting properties, such
as vitamins, minerals, and
antioxidants.

9. **Homeopathic Remedies:**

   - Homeopathic medicines are
     prepared from highly diluted plant
     extracts, following the principles
     of homeopathy. They are
     believed to stimulate the body's
     innate healing mechanisms and
     are used to treat a wide range of
     acute and chronic conditions.

10. **Herbal Steams and Inhalations:**

   - Herbal steams and inhalations
     involve inhaling steam infused

with medicinal plants or essential oils. They can help alleviate respiratory congestion, sinusitis, and promote respiratory health.

These are just a few examples of the diverse types of plant medicines available, each offering unique therapeutic benefits for supporting health and well-being.

Herbal Formulations and Applications

Herbal Formulations and Applications: Unlocking Nature's Healing Potentials

Herbal formulations and applications offer a myriad of ways to harness the therapeutic properties of medicinal plants for promoting health and well-being. From traditional remedies to modern formulations, explore the diverse world of herbal preparations and their practical applications in daily life.

Understanding Herbal Formulations:

- **Tinctures, Infusions, and Decoctions**: Learn the art of extracting medicinal compounds from herbs through various methods, including alcohol-based tinctures, water-based infusions, and simmered decoctions. Discover their unique properties, dosages, and applications for addressing different health concerns.
- **Topical Applications:** Explore the use of herbal salves, oils, poultices, and compresses for topical relief of skin

conditions, muscle soreness, joint pain, and wounds. Discover how herbal remedies can soothe inflammation, promote tissue regeneration, and enhance skin health when applied externally.

- **Internal Applications**: Delve into the world of herbal teas, tonics, elixirs, and capsules for internal use, offering systemic support for various bodily systems and functions. From enhancing digestion and immune function to supporting mental clarity and hormonal balance, herbal formulations provide versatile solutions for holistic wellness.

- **Cooking with Herbs:** Explore the culinary uses of medicinal plants and spices, adding flavor, nutrition, and therapeutic benefits to everyday meals. From herbal teas and infused oils to herbal soups, salads, and desserts, discover creative ways to incorporate herbs into your diet for vibrant health and culinary delight.

- **Herbal Skincare:** Discover the beauty-enhancing properties of botanical ingredients for nourishing and rejuvenating the skin. From herbal steam facials and masks to herbal-infused creams and serums, explore natural skincare routines that promote radiant complexion and overall skin health.

- **Self-Care Rituals:** Cultivate mindful self-care practices using herbal remedies to nurture your body, mind, and spirit. From herbal baths and foot soaks to aromatherapy blends and herbal meditation practices, learn how to create sacred rituals that promote relaxation, stress relief, and inner balance.

Empowerment Through Herbal Medicine:

- **Personalized Healing:** Embrace the art of herbal formulation to tailor remedies to your unique constitution, health needs, and preferences. By understanding the energetics, tastes, and actions of herbs, you can create personalized formulations that support your individual wellness journey.

- **Community Wellness:** Share the gift of herbal medicine with your community by offering herbal workshops, sharing recipes, and creating herbal products for friends and family. Cultivate a culture of empowerment and self-reliance as you inspire others to reconnect with nature's healing bounty.

Embark on a transformative journey of herbal formulations and applications, and unlock the healing potentials of nature's pharmacy for vibrant health and well-being. Whether you're blending herbal teas, crafting herbal skincare products, or creating herbal remedies for common ailments, embrace the wisdom of herbal medicine and discover the power of

plants to nourish, heal, and rejuvenate.

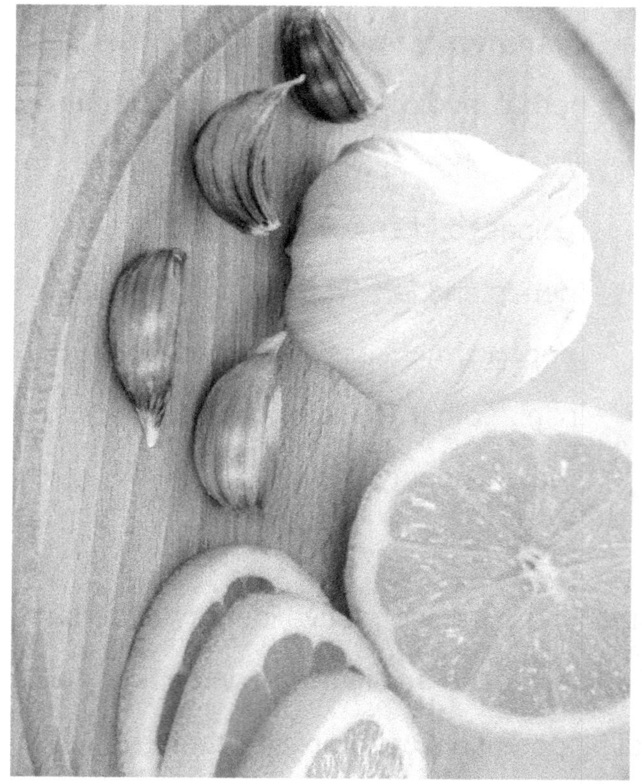

Chapter Five

Herbal Remedies for Common Ailments

Herbal remedies have been used for centuries to alleviate a wide range of common ailments, offering natural alternatives to conventional pharmaceuticals. Here's an extensive exploration of herbal remedies for some of the most prevalent health issues:

1. **Digestive Issues:**

- Peppermint (Mentha piperita): Relieves indigestion, bloating, and nausea by relaxing the muscles of the digestive tract.
- Ginger (Zingiber officinale): Aids digestion, reduces nausea, and alleviates stomach discomfort due to its anti-inflammatory and carminative properties.

- Chamomile (Matricaria chamomilla): Soothes stomach aches, promotes relaxation, and helps relieve symptoms of irritable bowel syndrome (IBS).

2. Respiratory Conditions:

- Eucalyptus (Eucalyptus globulus): Acts as a decongestant and expectorant, easing symptoms of coughs, colds, and sinus congestion.
- Thyme (Thymus vulgaris): Contains antimicrobial compounds that help fight respiratory infections, such as bronchitis and sore throats.
- Licorice root (Glycyrrhiza glabra): Soothes sore throats and coughs, and helps loosen mucus due to its demulcent and expectorant properties.

3. Stress and Anxiety:

- Ashwagandha (Withania somnifera): An adaptogenic herb that helps the body adapt to stress, promoting relaxation

and supporting overall mental
well-being.

- Holy Basil (Ocimum sanctum): Also
  known as Tulsi, it has calming and
  anti-anxiety effects, and helps improve
  resilience to stress.
- Lemon Balm (Melissa officinalis):
  Reduces anxiety, promotes relaxation,
  and improves sleep quality by
  increasing GABA levels in the brain.

4. **Sleep Disorders:**

- Valerian root (Valeriana officinalis): Acts
  as a sedative, promoting relaxation and
  improving sleep quality, particularly in
  cases of insomnia.
- Passionflower (Passiflora incarnata):
  Calms the nervous system, reduces
  anxiety, and aids in falling asleep and
  staying asleep.
- Lavender (Lavandula angustifolia):
  Induces relaxation, reduces insomnia,
  and promotes restful sleep when used
  as a tea or in aromatherapy.

5. Skin Conditions:

- Aloe Vera (Aloe barbadensis): Soothes burns, cuts, and minor wounds, and promotes skin healing due to its anti-inflammatory and moisturizing properties.
- Calendula (Calendula officinalis): Relieves skin inflammation, irritation, and minor infections, and accelerates wound healing.
- Tea Tree Oil (Melaleuca alternifolia): Exhibits antimicrobial and anti-inflammatory properties, making it effective against acne, fungal infections, and minor skin irritations.

6. Headaches and Migraines:

- Feverfew (Tanacetum parthenium): Reduces the frequency and severity of migraines by inhibiting inflammation and preventing blood vessel constriction.
- Butterbur (Petasites hybridus): Acts as a vasodilator and anti-inflammatory agent,

reducing the frequency and intensity of migraines.
- Willow Bark (Salix spp.): Contains salicin, a compound similar to aspirin, which relieves pain and inflammation associated with tension headaches and migraines.

7. Joint and Muscle Pain:

- Arnica (Arnica montana): Reduces inflammation, bruising, and muscle soreness, making it effective for treating injuries, sprains, and arthritis.
- Turmeric (Curcuma longa): Exhibits anti-inflammatory and analgesic properties, relieving pain and stiffness associated with osteoarthritis and rheumatoid arthritis.
- Devil's Claw (Harpagophytum procumbens): Acts as a natural pain reliever and anti-inflammatory agent, particularly beneficial for arthritis and muscle pain.

8. Immune Support:

- Echinacea (Echinacea purpurea): Boosts the immune system and reduces the severity and duration of colds and upper respiratory infections.
- Astragalus (Astragalus membranaceus): Enhances immune function, increases resistance to infections, and reduces the frequency of colds and flu.
- Elderberry (Sambucus nigra): Exhibits antiviral properties and supports immune function, reducing the severity and duration of colds and flu.

9. Diabetes:

- Gymnema (Gymnema sylvestre): Helps regulate blood sugar levels by stimulating insulin production and improving insulin sensitivity.
- Fenugreek (Trigonella foenum-graecum): Reduces blood glucose levels, improves insulin sensitivity, and helps lower cholesterol levels.
- Bitter Melon (Momordica charantia): Contains compounds that mimic insulin,

helping to lower blood sugar levels and improve glucose tolerance.

10. Hypertension:

- Hawthorn (Crataegus spp.): Dilates blood vessels, improves blood flow, and lowers blood pressure due to its antioxidant and anti-inflammatory properties.
- Garlic (Allium sativum): Acts as a vasodilator, reduces blood pressure, and improves circulation by inhibiting platelet aggregation and cholesterol synthesis.
- Olive Leaf (Olea europaea): Lowers blood pressure and improves heart health by relaxing blood vessels and reducing inflammation.

11. Menstrual Disorders:

- Chaste Tree (Vitex agnus-castus): Regulates menstrual cycles, reduces PMS symptoms, and alleviates

symptoms of menopause by balancing hormones.
- Dong Quai (Angelica sinensis): Relieves menstrual cramps, regulates menstrual flow, and balances hormone levels, particularly estrogen.
- Black Cohosh (Actaea racemosa): Eases menstrual discomfort, reduces hot flashes, and relieves symptoms of menopause by modulating hormone levels.

These herbal remedies offer safe and effective alternatives for managing common ailments, but it's essential to consult with a qualified healthcare practitioner before using them, especially if you have any underlying health conditions or are taking medications. Additionally, individual responses to herbal remedies may vary, so it's crucial to monitor for any adverse reactions and adjust usage accordingly.

The Science Behind plant medicine

The science behind plant medicine, often referred to as phytotherapy or phytomedicine, encompasses a diverse range of disciplines, including pharmacology, biochemistry, botany, and traditional medicine. This interdisciplinary field explores the therapeutic properties of plants and their bioactive compounds, shedding light on the mechanisms of action and potential applications in healthcare. Here's an overview of the science behind plant medicine:

1. **Identification and Characterization of Bioactive Compounds:**
   - Scientists analyze plant materials to identify and characterize

bioactive compounds responsible
for their medicinal properties.
This involves techniques such as
chromatography, spectroscopy,
and mass spectrometry.

- Compounds like alkaloids,
  flavonoids, terpenes, and
  phenolic compounds are among
  the many bioactive constituents
  found in medicinal plants.

2. Pharmacological Research and Mechanisms of Action:

- Pharmacological studies
  investigate how plant compounds
  interact with biological systems to
  produce therapeutic effects. This
  includes studying their effects on
  receptors, enzymes, and
  signaling pathways.

- o Understanding the mechanisms
  of action helps elucidate how
  plant medicines exert their effects
  on specific health conditions,
  such as anti-inflammatory,
  antioxidant, or antimicrobial
  activity.

3. **Clinical Trials and Evidence-Based Medicine:**

   - o Clinical trials assess the safety
     and efficacy of plant-based
     treatments in human subjects.
     These studies provide scientific
     evidence to support the use of
     plant medicines for various health
     conditions.

   - o Randomized controlled trials
     (RCTs), systematic reviews, and
     meta-analyses contribute to

evidence-based medicine,
guiding healthcare practitioners in
the selection and use of
plant-based therapies.

4. **Phytochemical Pharmacokinetics and Pharmacodynamics:**

   - Phytochemical pharmacokinetics examines the absorption, distribution, metabolism, and excretion of plant compounds in the body. This helps determine optimal dosages and treatment regimens.

   - Pharmacodynamics explores how plant compounds exert their effects at the molecular, cellular, and physiological levels, elucidating their impact on disease processes and health outcomes.

5. **Drug Discovery and Development:**

    - Plant-derived compounds serve as valuable sources for drug discovery and development. Pharmaceutical companies screen plant extracts and isolated compounds for potential therapeutic applications.

    - Natural products have yielded numerous drugs used in modern medicine, including aspirin (from willow bark), morphine (from opium poppy), and quinine (from cinchona bark).

6. **Phytotherapy Integration with Conventional Medicine:**

- Integrative medicine combines conventional treatments with evidence-based complementary therapies, including phytotherapy. This approach enhances patient care by addressing the root causes of illness and promoting holistic well-being.
- Healthcare providers collaborate to ensure safe and effective integration of plant-based medicines with conventional treatments, taking into account individual patient needs and preferences.

7. **Herbal Quality Control and Standardization:**

- Quality control measures ensure the safety, purity, and consistency

of herbal products. This includes
authentication of plant species,
testing for contaminants, and
standardization of active
ingredients.

- Regulatory agencies establish
  guidelines and standards for the
  manufacturing, labeling, and
  marketing of herbal supplements
  and botanical medicines to
  protect public health.

The science behind plant medicine continues
to evolve, driven by ongoing research,
technological advancements, and a growing
appreciation for the therapeutic potential of
natural remedies. Through rigorous scientific
inquiry, plant medicine bridges the gap
between traditional healing practices and

modern healthcare, offering safe, effective, and evidence-based solutions for promoting health and well-being.

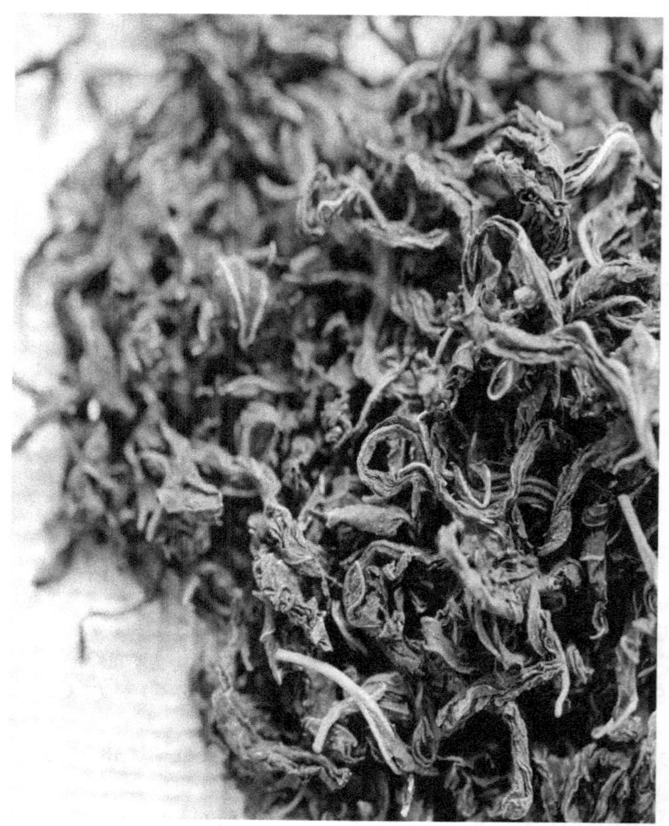

Chapter Six

Cultivating A Medicinal Garden

Cultivating a medicinal garden is a fulfilling and practical endeavor that allows individuals to connect with nature while nurturing a diverse array of plants with therapeutic properties. Whether you have a small backyard, a balcony, or even just a sunny windowsill, creating a medicinal garden can provide a sustainable source of herbal remedies and enhance your overall well-being. Here's a guide to cultivating your own medicinal garden:

1. **Selecting the Right Location:**

- Choose a location with ample sunlight, as most medicinal plants require direct sunlight for healthy growth. Ensure the area has good drainage to prevent waterlogging, which can cause root rot.

- Consider factors such as proximity to water sources, protection from strong winds, and accessibility for regular maintenance and harvesting.

2. Designing Your Garden Layout:

- Plan your garden layout based on the space available and the specific needs of the plants you intend to grow. Think about combining plants that need the same amount of sunshine and water.
- Incorporate features such as raised beds, containers, or trellises to maximize space and create visual interest in your garden.

3. **Choosing Medicinal Plants:**

- Research different medicinal plants and select species that are well-suited to your climate, soil type, and growing conditions. Consider both native and non-native species, but prioritize plants that are adapted to your local environment.
- Choose a variety of plants with different therapeutic properties, such as herbs for digestion, immune support, stress relief, and skin care.

4. **Preparing the Soil:**

- Test the soil pH and fertility levels to determine if any amendments are needed. Most medicinal plants prefer well-draining soil with a slightly acidic to neutral pH.

- Incorporate organic matter such as compost, aged manure, or leaf mulch to improve soil structure, fertility, and moisture retention.

5. **Planting and Maintenance:**

- Follow planting instructions specific to each plant, including spacing, depth, and watering requirements. Plant seeds or seedlings according to the recommended spacing and depth.
- Water newly planted seedlings regularly to establish strong root systems. Once established, most medicinal plants require moderate watering, allowing the soil to dry out between waterings.

- Mulch around plants to suppress weeds, retain moisture, and regulate soil temperature. Monitor for pests and diseases regularly and take appropriate measures to control them using organic methods whenever possible.

6. Harvesting and Preserving Medicinal Plants:

- Familiarize yourself with the optimal time to harvest each plant part (leaves, flowers, roots, etc.) for maximum potency and efficacy. When essential oils are at their most concentrated in the morning, harvest.
- Dry herbs and plant materials thoroughly before storing them to prevent mold and spoilage. Use

methods such as air drying, dehydrating, or hanging bundles in a well-ventilated area.

- Store dried herbs in airtight containers away from light, heat, and moisture to maintain their potency and flavor. Label containers with the plant name and date of harvest for easy identification.

7. **Continuing Education and Experimentation:**

- Stay curious and continue learning about different medicinal plants, their therapeutic properties, and how to use them effectively. Explore herbal books, online resources, workshops, and gardening clubs for inspiration and knowledge sharing.

- Experiment with different growing techniques, companion planting strategies, and herbal preparations to find what works best for your garden and your health needs.

Cultivating a medicinal garden is a rewarding journey that fosters a deeper connection with nature while empowering you to take control of your health and well-being. Whether you're a seasoned gardener or a novice, the process of growing, harvesting, and using medicinal plants can enrich your life and enhance your relationship with the natural world.

DIY Plant Medicine Recipes

Certainly! Here are some simple do-it-yourself (DIY) plant medicine recipes that you can make at home using common medicinal herbs and ingredients:

1. Herbal Tea Blend for Immune Support:

- Ingredients:
    1. 1 part dried echinacea root
    2. 1 part dried elderberries
    3. 1 part dried ginger root
- Instructions:
    1. Combine the dried herbs in a mixing bowl, ensuring equal parts of each.
    2. Store the blend in an airtight container.

3. To prepare, steep 1 tablespoon of the herbal blend in 8 ounces of hot water for 10-15 minutes. Strain and enjoy. Drink 2-3 cups daily for immune support during cold and flu season.

2. Calming Lavender Bath Salts:

- Ingredients:
    1. 1 cup Epsom salt
    2. ¼ cup dried lavender flowers
    3. 10-15 drops lavender essential oil
- Instructions:
    1. In a mixing bowl, combine the Epsom salt and dried lavender flowers.

2. In order to properly disperse the smell, add the lavender essential oil and stir well.

3. To store the mixture, transfer it to a jar that is clean and airtight.

4. To use, add ½ cup of the lavender bath salts to a warm bath and soak for 20-30 minutes to relax the body and calm the mind.

3. Herbal Salve for Skin Healing:

- Ingredients:
    1. ½ cup infused herbal oil (e.g., calendula, comfrey, or plantain)
    2. 2 tablespoons beeswax pellets

3. Optional: 10-15 drops of essential oils (e.g., lavender, tea tree, or chamomile)

- Instructions:

   1. Melt the beeswax pellets at low heat in a double boiler.

   2. Once melted, add the infused herbal oil and stir until well combined.

   3. Remove from heat and let the mixture cool slightly.

   4. If using essential oils, add them to the mixture and stir well.

   5. Pour the mixture into clean, sterilized containers (e.g., jars or tins) and let it cool and solidify before sealing.

   6. Apply the herbal salve topically to minor cuts, scrapes, burns, or dry

skin as needed for healing and soothing relief.

4. Digestive Bitters Tincture:

- Ingredients:
    1. 1 part dried dandelion root
    2. 1 part dried gentian root
    3. 1 part dried fennel seeds
    4. 1 part dried orange peel
    5. 80-proof vodka or brandy
- Instructions:
    1. Combine the dried herbs in a clean, sterilized glass jar, filling it halfway.
    2. Pour enough alcohol over the herbs to completely cover them, ensuring they are fully submerged.

3. Seal the jar tightly and store it in a cool, dark place for 4-6 weeks, shaking it daily to ensure thorough extraction.

4. After the steeping period, strain the tincture through cheesecloth or a fine mesh sieve into a clean glass dropper bottle.

5. Label the bottle with the tincture name and date of preparation.

6. To use, take 1-2 dropperfuls of the digestive bitters tincture diluted in a small amount of water before meals to support digestion and stimulate digestive juices.

These DIY plant medicine recipes offer simple and effective ways to incorporate herbal remedies into your daily routine for health and well-being. Experiment with different herbs and ingredients to create personalized remedies tailored to your specific needs and preferences.

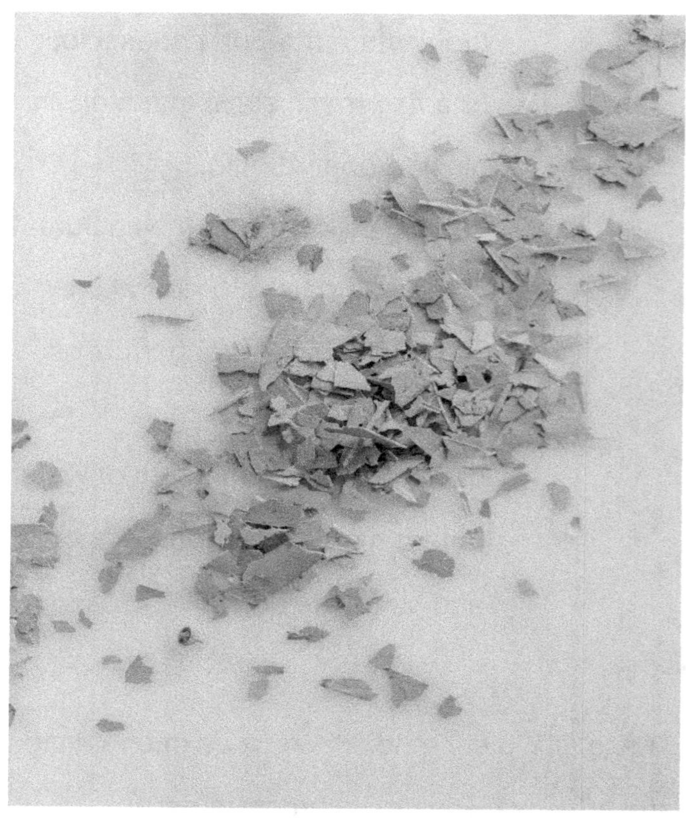

Chapter Seven

Responsible Use and Safety

Responsible use and safety are paramount when it comes to utilizing plant medicine. While natural remedies can offer numerous health benefits, it's essential to approach their use with caution and respect for both the plants and your own well-being. Here are some guidelines for responsibly using and ensuring safety with plant medicine:

1. **Educate Yourself:**

- Before using any plant-based remedy, educate yourself about its properties, potential side effects, and contraindications. Research reputable sources, consult herbal books, or seek

guidance from qualified healthcare
professionals or herbalists.

2. Start Slowly:

- When trying a new herbal remedy, start
  with a low dose and gradually increase it
  as needed. This allows you to gauge
  your body's response and tolerance to
  the plant's effects.

3. Know Your Body:

- Pay attention to how your body
  responds to herbal remedies. If you feel
  uncomfortable or have any negative
  reactions, stop using the product and
  see a doctor.

4. **Quality Matters:**

- Choose high-quality, organically grown herbs from reputable sources to ensure purity and potency. Avoid using plants that may have been exposed to pesticides, heavy metals, or other contaminants.

5. **Respect Dosages:**

- Follow recommended dosages and usage instructions carefully. Overconsumption of certain plants or herbal preparations can lead to adverse effects or toxicity.

6. **Be Mindful of Interactions:**

- Be aware of potential interactions between herbal remedies and medications you may be taking. Some plants can interact with prescription drugs, affecting their efficacy or causing adverse reactions.

7. Use Caution During Pregnancy and Lactation:

- Exercise caution when using herbal remedies during pregnancy and breastfeeding, as some plants may have adverse effects on fetal development or infant health. Consult a healthcare professional before using any herbal products during these times.

8. Perform Patch Tests:

- Before using herbal remedies topically, such as herbal salves or essential oils, perform a patch test on a small area of skin to check for allergic reactions or sensitivities.

9. Store Safely:

- Store herbal products in a cool, dry place away from direct sunlight and moisture to maintain their potency and freshness. Make sure that dogs and youngsters cannot access them.

10. Practice Sustainable Harvesting:

- If harvesting plants from the wild, do so responsibly and sustainably. Avoid overharvesting and only collect plants from areas where they are abundant and legal to harvest. Respect indigenous peoples' rights and cultural practices related to plant harvesting.

11. Seek Professional Guidance:

- Consult with a qualified healthcare professional or herbalist, especially if you have pre-existing health conditions, are pregnant or breastfeeding, or are unsure about using certain herbs. They can provide personalized guidance and ensure safe and effective use of plant medicine.

By following these guidelines for responsible use and safety, you can enjoy the benefits of plant medicine while minimizing risks and promoting overall well-being. Remember that every individual is unique, and what works well for one person may not be suitable for another. Listen to your body, trust your instincts, and prioritize safety in your journey with plant-based remedies.

Legal And Ethical Considerations

Legal and ethical considerations are essential aspects to be mindful of when it comes to the use of plant medicine. While natural remedies have been used for centuries, navigating the legal landscape and adhering to ethical principles ensures the safe and responsible utilization of plant-based therapies. The

following are important legal and moral things
to remember:

1. Regulatory Compliance:

- Familiarize yourself with the regulatory
  framework governing herbal products
  and supplements in your region or
  country. Laws and regulations may vary
  regarding the cultivation, sale, labeling,
  and marketing of herbal remedies.
- Ensure that any herbal products you
  purchase or sell comply with relevant
  regulations, including Good
  Manufacturing Practices (GMP) and
  labeling requirements.

2. Quality and Safety Standards:

- Prioritize the use of high-quality, ethically sourced herbs and botanical ingredients. Choose reputable suppliers that adhere to quality and safety standards, such as organic certification and sustainable harvesting practices.
- Conduct thorough research and due diligence to verify the authenticity and purity of herbal products, especially if purchasing from online or international sources.

3. Informed Consent and Disclosure:

- Provide clear and accurate information to consumers about the potential benefits, risks, and limitations of herbal remedies. Ensure that individuals are fully informed before using herbal products and obtain their informed consent.

- Disclose any known contraindications, interactions with medications, or potential side effects associated with herbal remedies to promote transparency and empower consumers to make informed decisions about their health.

4. Cultural Respect and Indigenous Rights:

- Acknowledge and respect indigenous peoples' cultural knowledge, traditional healing practices, and intellectual property rights associated with medicinal plants. Avoid appropriating or exploiting indigenous knowledge without proper acknowledgment or consent.

- Collaborate with indigenous communities in a respectful and equitable manner, honoring their sovereignty, autonomy, and ancestral connections to the land and plant medicines.

5. Environmental Sustainability:

- Practice sustainable harvesting and cultivation methods to ensure the long-term viability of medicinal plant populations and ecosystems. Avoid overharvesting, habitat destruction, and exploitation of endangered or threatened species.
- Support initiatives and organizations dedicated to conservation, biodiversity protection, and sustainable wildcrafting

practices, contributing to the preservation of medicinal plants for future generations.

6. Professional Ethics and Scope of Practice:

- If you are a healthcare practitioner or herbalist, adhere to ethical guidelines and professional standards of practice when recommending or prescribing herbal remedies. Respect the boundaries of your expertise and refer clients to qualified professionals when appropriate.
- Maintain client confidentiality, uphold professional integrity, and prioritize the well-being and autonomy of individuals seeking herbal healthcare services.

7. Community Engagement and Education:

- Foster community engagement and education about the safe and responsible use of herbal remedies. Provide accessible resources, workshops, and educational materials to empower individuals to make informed choices about their health.
- Promote cultural diversity, inclusivity, and equity within herbalism, recognizing the contributions of diverse cultures and perspectives to the field of plant medicine.

By adhering to these legal and ethical considerations, individuals and practitioners can navigate the complexities of plant medicine responsibly, fostering a culture of safety, integrity, and sustainability in the use of herbal remedies for health and well-being.

Herb

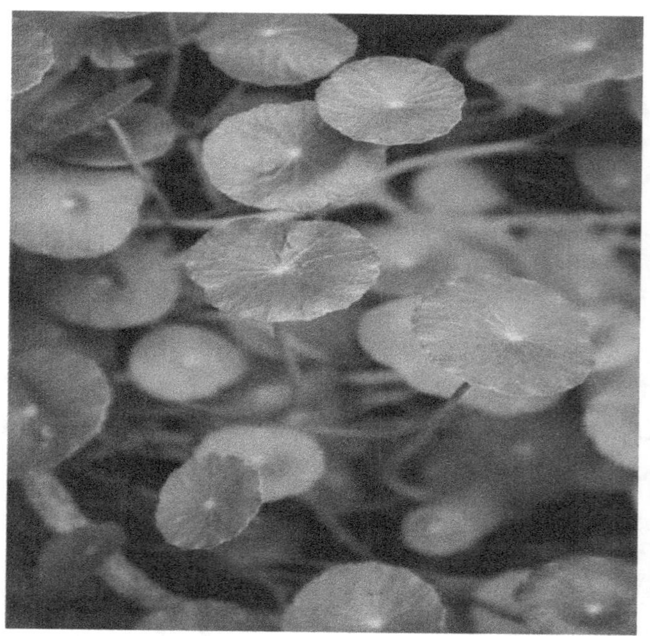

Chapter Eight

The Future of Plant Medicine

The future of plant medicine is poised to be dynamic and transformative, driven by advancements in scientific research, technological innovation, and a growing appreciation for the therapeutic potential of natural remedies. Here are some key trends and developments shaping the future of plant medicine:

1. Integration of Traditional Knowledge with Modern Science:

- There is a growing recognition of the value of traditional knowledge systems and indigenous practices in plant medicine. Integrating ancient wisdom with modern scientific methods allows for a more holistic understanding of plant remedies and their effects on human health.

- Collaborative research initiatives between indigenous communities, scientists, and healthcare professionals facilitate the documentation, validation, and preservation of traditional herbal knowledge, ensuring its continued relevance and accessibility.

2. **Personalized and Precision Herbal Medicine:**

- Advances in genomics, metabolomics, and personalized medicine are paving the way for personalized herbal therapies tailored to individual genetic makeup, health status, and lifestyle factors.

- Precision herbal medicine involves identifying biomarkers, genetic variations, and other factors that influence an individual's response to herbal remedies, allowing for targeted interventions and optimized treatment outcomes.

3. Pharmacological and Mechanistic Insights:

- Ongoing pharmacological research is unraveling the mechanisms of action underlying the therapeutic effects of plant compounds. This deeper understanding of bioactive constituents and their interactions with biological

targets informs the development of
novel herbal formulations and
therapeutic strategies.

- Pharmacogenomic studies elucidate
genetic variations that influence drug
metabolism and response, providing
insights into personalized dosing
regimens and potential drug-herb
interactions.

4. Innovations in Herbal Formulations and Delivery Systems:

- Technological innovations such as
nanoencapsulation, liposomal delivery,
and phytochemical complexation
enhance the bioavailability, stability, and
efficacy of herbal extracts and
phytochemicals.

- Novel formulations such as herbal nanoparticles, micelles, and emulsions enable targeted delivery of plant compounds to specific tissues or organs, optimizing therapeutic outcomes and minimizing side effects.

5. Plant-Based Therapies for Chronic Diseases:

- Plant medicine is increasingly recognized as a valuable adjunct or alternative therapy for managing chronic diseases such as diabetes, cardiovascular disorders, autoimmune conditions, and neurodegenerative diseases.
- Clinical trials and epidemiological studies support the efficacy of certain

herbal remedies in improving metabolic health, reducing inflammation, modulating immune function, and enhancing neuroprotection.

6. Sustainability and Conservation Initiatives:

- With growing concerns about biodiversity loss, habitat destruction, and overharvesting of medicinal plants, there is a greater emphasis on sustainable cultivation, wildcrafting practices, and conservation efforts.
- Initiatives such as fair trade certification, organic farming practices, and community-based stewardship programs promote ethical sourcing, equitable trade relations, and

environmental stewardship in the herbal industry.

7. Public Education and Awareness:

- Increasing public awareness about the benefits of plant medicine, coupled with demand for natural and holistic healthcare options, drives the popularity and acceptance of herbal remedies.
- Educational initiatives, online resources, and integrative healthcare models empower individuals to take an active role in their health and well-being, fostering a culture of self-care, prevention, and empowerment.

In summary, the future of plant medicine holds tremendous promise for revolutionizing healthcare, with a focus on personalized, evidence-based approaches that honor the rich legacy of traditional healing practices while embracing the opportunities afforded by modern science and technology. By harnessing the therapeutic potential of plants in a sustainable, ethical, and inclusive manner, plant medicine has the potential to contribute to a healthier, more resilient, and interconnected world.

Conclusion

In conclusion, herbal medicine offers a rich tapestry of remedies for addressing a wide range of health conditions, from common ailments to specific disorders. With a history spanning millennia and rooted in diverse cultural traditions, herbalism embodies the timeless wisdom of harnessing nature's healing power.

The extensive exploration of herbal remedies provided highlights the breadth and depth of herbal medicine's therapeutic potential. Whether it's relieving digestive issues, managing chronic conditions like diabetes and hypertension, or supporting mental health and immune function, herbal remedies offer safe and effective alternatives to conventional pharmaceuticals.

Furthermore, herbal medicine promotes a holistic approach to health, recognizing the interconnectedness of mind, body, and spirit. By addressing underlying imbalances and supporting the body's innate healing capacity, herbal remedies not only alleviate symptoms but also promote overall well-being and vitality.

However, it's essential to approach herbal medicine with caution and respect, consulting qualified healthcare practitioners and considering individual needs and circumstances. While herbal remedies are generally considered safe when used appropriately, they can interact with medications and may not be suitable for everyone.

In today's rapidly evolving healthcare landscape, herbal medicine continues to

inspire hope and healing, offering a bridge
between ancient wisdom and modern science.
As we navigate the complexities of health and
wellness, embracing the principles of herbalism
can empower us to cultivate resilience, foster
connection with nature, and embark on a
journey towards holistic health and harmony.
Additionally, the resurgence of interest in
herbal medicine reflects a growing recognition
of the importance of sustainability,
environmental stewardship, and cultural
preservation. By promoting the cultivation of
medicinal plants, supporting local growers, and
advocating for ethical wildcrafting practices,
herbalism fosters a deeper connection to the
Earth and promotes biodiversity.

As we continue to explore the potential of
herbal medicine, it's crucial to integrate
traditional knowledge with modern scientific

research, ensuring evidence-based practices and informed decision-making. Collaborative efforts between herbalists, researchers, and healthcare professionals can further advance our understanding of medicinal plants and their therapeutic applications.

In essence, herbal medicine embodies a holistic approach to health and healing, honoring the innate wisdom of nature and celebrating the interconnectedness of all living beings. By embracing herbalism, we not only embark on a journey towards optimal health but also cultivate a deeper sense of connection, resilience, and harmony with the natural world. As we navigate the complexities of modern life, let us draw inspiration from the healing power of plants and embark on a path of wellness guided by the timeless principles of herbal medicine.